The Sport of Happiness

Learn to Experience Joy,
Even When You Don't Feel Happy

Written By: Iasha King

Contents

INTRODUCTION

"Play to win" - Iasha (author and girl who lost more times than she can count)

Have you ever laid in bed at 3 am thinking "Who decided the alphabet was in alphabetical order?" Well, you may not have had that exact thought, but I swear, 1 am- 4 am are when some of the deepest thoughts come into your mind. Forget about work; you now have to contemplate how you would describe the taste of water to someone who never had it.

I began having restless sleep due to my thoughts shortly after college. One day I got to the point where I was sick and tired, of being sick and tired. I knew I wanted more in life and was discouraged at how my life was going at that point. I was 25 going on 50 it felt like. Not that there's anything wrong with being 50 years old, but damn where did the time go? One moment I'm living it up studying abroad, moving to Hawaii, meeting new people, to then staring at the wall every weekend (okay it wasn't that bad, but things did kind of suck).

Anytime something went wrong I would become this ball of anger. That anger from one day would then seep into future days. Sadness came with anger and happiness only felt possible if good things would happen. Like most people, my happiness depended on my circumstances. It took me quite a bit of time to change my behavior and thoughts towards happiness. I hope to share these life-transforming revelations with you!

I've been a competitive athlete for more than 15 years and have lived and breathed sports my whole life. I have been coached and mentored by some amazing human beings. I know first-hand the importance of having an actionable plan. I could hope all day to win a gold medal but if I didn't have a plan on how to get there then it would never happen. I also know how special it is to have a coach help guide you on your journey.

This book is called "The Sport of Happiness" in order for you to understand that reaching your goal of living a life of joy takes practice and a plan. Like any athlete, you will need discipline, perseverance, drive, and confidence for long-lasting effects. Athletes such as Serena Williams, Michael Phelps, and Manny Pacquiao did not become top performers in their sport in mere months. Exercising habits of happiness may take weeks or months before you really start to feel the difference.

Happiness is an emotional state we find ourselves in due to external factors. When we eat a yummy meal, find money, ace a test, get a new job, we experience a feeling of happiness. But what happens when those 'happy moments' don't come every day? Practicing happiness habits will help us in being in a long-term state of joy, rather than a temporary state of happiness. You will commit to not only practicing happiness when we feel like it but just like an athlete, practice even when you don't want to.

At the beginning of building these happiness habits, you may feel like a fraud. Imposter syndrome is real. However, like any habit, happiness will start to feel like a natural state of being. You will see the benefits in many ways that you never expected. Joyful people have better relationships, happier work lives, and overall better aurora. You may even walk past those people and dread their cheerfulness. Don't hate, just join the team.

Joyful people come in all shapes and sizes with their own quirks. I'm not talking about being happy when happiness is due. I'm talking about being a person who is at ease with themselves and has a genuine love of life. Therefore, no need to change your wardrobe and buy 'hippie clothing', no need to paint your house yellow to represent eternal sunshine, and you don't have to buy a guitar to learn how to play 'Kumbaya' at the first bonfire you see. There is no stereotype of what a joyful person looks like.

You may start to see changes in your behavior and thoughts, and that is okay, great even if it leads to a healthier and happier you. This happiness journey is about you becoming the best version of yourself. And only you know what that looks like.

CH 1: FEELINGS ARE TRICKY

"Just because you feel tired,
doesn't mean you are tired"

One of my favorite athletic training stories comes from the inspirational David Goggins, a retired Navy SEAL Chief, author, motivational speaker, and overall badass. He is often called the 'Toughest Man Alive' for his ability to overcome obstacle after obstacle using both mental and physical strength that most people can never imagine. At a certain point in his life, David realized he wanted to do something that would challenge him and hopefully help break him to be something greater. Days before the famous Badwater Ultramarathon-135-mile race in California, David entered, never having run anything close to 100 miles before in his life. I personally would have assumed there was a typo and show up thinking we're about to run 10 miles, but not his guy. He left the race having finished in 19 hours. But the most memorable part was not him finishing the race, but what he endured in order to cross the finish line.

This ultramarathon was in the valley during the summer. Already you can imagine how difficult this would be especially due to the heat at just one mile. In order to even qualify for this race, he had to first prove he could finish 100 miles in 24 hours or less. Now remember David had never run 100 miles before, and I myself would have cried thinking it was supposed to be 10.

At mile 70 he sat down and thought to himself "This is it, there is no way I can go on". His feeling of tiredness wasn't the normal "Oh I only had 4 hours of sleep, how am I going to make it through work and go to the gym today". This feeling of tiredness was extreme. Most people would have advised him to stop given his injuries at that point. However, he was so driven to complete this race, that he ended up pushing through all of his pain and completing the race in the allotted amount of time. He spent 19 grueling hours running in circles on a track limping home with stress fractures, shin splints, and muscle tears...but he did it.

No one in the world likes feeling "Got". No one wants to feel like they've been tricked or swindled, yet that's exactly what <u>feelings</u> can do to us every day. Although feelings give us a great insight into what state of mind we are in and how we react to external situations, they never really give us the full picture. In some ways, feelings can act as protection and keep us from harm's way. I'm sure you've heard stories of people attributing their survival to intuition. How they sensed danger, felt something was off/wrong, and ended up avoiding a devastating situation. Or you may have come into a situation yourself where you encountered a person and you just didn't feel right so you decided to get away from them (something just ain't right with people who purposefully eat warm potato salad).

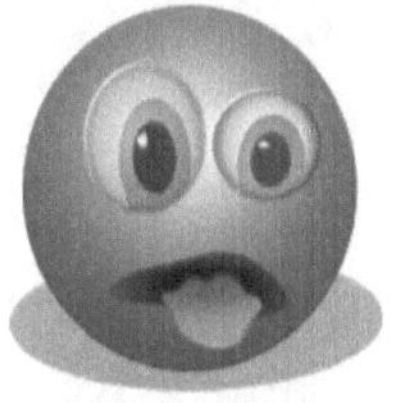

Feelings can also help us decipher our own biases towards people and situations. Our feelings change as situations change. This is why it is important to note the fragility of feelings as a whole. It is a reminder for us to think about those feelings when they arise, and ask ourselves "Why do I feel this way"? Think of feeling like a process. The sensation of feeling arising is just the beginning. You should never stop there. You should never start to feel something and think, "This feeling is going to last and it's who I am now".

For most of us, if we allowed feelings to dictate our lives, our lives would seem darker than they really are. For some reason, we as humans tend to dwell on the negatives. It's amazing how something as small as getting cut off in traffic can ruin our whole day. We think about it while someone holds the elevator for us, we fume over it while we eat lunch with our friends, and obsess over it while eating a meal a loved one cooked for us. We allow these negative thoughts to consume us, which keeps us from enjoying the other positive things going on in our lives.

After that person cuts you off in traffic, you may have felt anger. Does that mean you're angry now? If so, for how long? You may be angry, but another person can be cut off by the same driver down the road and feel essentially nothing. We have to learn and truly understand that feelings are subjective and always changing. Therefore, we cannot accept them as they are at face value. If a math teacher says $2 + 2 = 4$ we understand that yes that is true, there is no denying that. However, it wouldn't be necessarily right to say "This person made me feel angry, and now I AM angry". We can feel something arising without allowing it to manifest. We are going to start doing something else, just be patient.

Our feelings do not have to define our state of mind for the rest of the day, month, or year. There should be freedom and hope in knowing that your state of living does not depend on external factors. Feelings arise, sometimes unconsciously, but then we always have the choice to continue to feel that way or not. This of course is not always easy for people, especially for those experiencing the effects of mental health problems or experiencing extreme hardships. For those people, happiness exercises may be more challenging to start, but with the right drive and team behind you (including ME!!), I'm confident that your joy journey will be just as successful.

Practicing happiness requires us to first acknowledge that feelings are temporary. They do not dictate our long-term state of being (mentally and physically). Once we understand this, we can start to control how we react to our feelings and how we perceive them. This in turn allows us to eventually start to implement the short-term and long-term habits for an immediate feeling of happiness that leads to long-lasting joy.

CH 2: PAIN & PERSPECTIVE

Life can be very painful. Anger does not always arise from something small such as someone cutting you off in traffic. Sometimes your feeling of anger can arise from something greater. Factors beyond our control can affect how we feel. Our pain can come from natural disasters, disease, accidents, or at the hands of other people. Pain is also subjective, which is in part due to your perspective and tolerance.

Pain and tragedy are real. I believe no one should be able to tell you how and when to feel. No one likes to be belittled or told their problems are insignificant. The journey of changing perspective is a personal one. Tragedies such as losing a loved one, suffering from sickness, being a victim of a crime, often warrant feelings of sadness, anger, and possibly guilt. You deserve time to mourn and which hopefully leads to a path of healing. There can be no hope of healing if you never release those emotions you may be holding in.

Learning to see things from a different perspective will not always stop pain from entering our lives. It is not to downplay your troubles. That habit of changing your perspective deals with your ability to practice empathy and gratitude. Everyone can use a little more empathy and gratitude no matter where you are on your joy journey.

I remember talking to my childhood friend one day who was talking about how upset she was over losing $75 out of her pocket the previous night. She went on to explain how she was thinking about it while she was trying to go to sleep, and how she didn't want to go out with friends since she was still "pissed". This is a financially successful friend in my book who makes 6-figures a year in the medical field and who owns a home. At the same time, I was unemployed and temporarily moved back to my parents' home to get back on my feet. In the back of my head I'm thinking, "$75 in the grand scheme of things isn't nothing, I'm the one who should be pissed, I don't have any income".

Isn't it funny how we frown upon people who complain who "have it good", without realizing we may have it good ourselves? Some could look at my situation and say "At least you had a home to go to". While someone else could look at that person and say "At least you're healthy". We can always find someone else hurting more than we are. However, it is not healthy or important to compare your situation with someone else. Comparing yourself to other people is a bad habit to make. Just like your fingerprint, there is no one like you so why compare yourself?

Simultaneously, it may be just as difficult for a person who is struggling to find joy at their job as a person experiencing houselessness to feel gratitude. It depends on the person, their upbringing, and beliefs. It is important to understand that our situations have no bearing on our ability to practice gratitude. Have you ever wondered why people in some of the poorest countries seem happier than those in the wealthiest parts? It's about being content with where you are in that moment and grateful for the opportunity to be alive.

Some people go to extremes to feel the joy of what simply living brings. I've heard of wealthy business professionals leaving their corporate jobs to pursue something they're passionate about. Sometimes this means sacrificing their cushiony lifestyle and living very modestly. Another great example is the allure behind people backpacking around the world. Traveling the world can be an expensive feat but one of the most eye-opening experiences one could ever have. People have found creative ways to fund this lifetime adventure and with bare minimal material things, they set off to learn and experience life outside of their comfort zone. This sometimes requires people to live in temporary and modest housing, ration on food, and get lost in unknown cities (plenty of getting lost). But the opportunity to simply live and learn and experience life makes it all worth it.

Currently, we are in the midst of a global pandemic that hit every country on earth in 2020. As businesses shut down all around the world, people had to adapt to staying home more. Yay introverts boohoo extroverts. I at times would find myself bored out of my mind. But I remember thinking one day, "I have a TV, cable, all the subscription TV channels you can think of, books, a kindle, laptop, internet, phone, free international calling, and yet I'm still bored!" I had to check myself and put myself in a place of gratefulness. At a time where thousands of people were dying every day, I was able to stay relatively healthy. I'm also sure I had way more 'entertainment' resources at my disposal than other people around the world. Although quarantine may have not been the most social environment, many people took that time to grow, learn, and transform themselves. It all goes back to perspective.

CH 3: HAPPINESS VS. JOY

"Choosing happiness consistently
will lead to joy"

Some of my favorite things to listen to are motivation videos, whether that be podcasts, Youtube videos, speeches, etc. I love hearing about people's stories and how they achieved the impossible and made it out a success. The sad truth is not all of us will become millionaires, homeowners, business entrepreneurs, or a celebrity. Hell, not everyone wants to even be any of those things. However, for those who do, that thought and the inability to achieve it now is oftentimes what is keeping joy from entering our life. In this example, your happiness is based solely on your achievements.

While joy and happiness are often used interchangeably, they are fundamentally different. Your feeling of happiness depends on external factors such as people, events, and things. While joy is said to be of an internal state of being. It is more consistent and dependent upon you.

While feeling happy is a good thing, it shouldn't be our end goal. The problem with relying on feeling happy is that we have to wait on somebody or something else to make it happen. So, what do we do/feel in between that time? In this book, we will often describe the journey as taking small steps every day. These small steps are in the form of exercises that make you feel better at that moment. Then as these habits become daily behaviors and thoughts, you then start to find yourself in a longer state of joy.

The act of practicing happiness lies in the action of choosing happiness every day. It is important to make small every day conscious decisions to be happy. This mindset is just as important as doing physical tricks to make you feel happy.

CH 4: EMBRACE THE SUCK

Bethany Hamilton is a professional surfer who has had massive success on and off the water. You may have read her book *"Soul Surfer: A True Story of Faith, Family, and Fighting to Get Back on the Board"* or watched her movie *"Soul Surfer"* highlighting her inspiring career. In 2003, Bethany survived a shark attack which consequently led to her losing her left arm. Despite the tragic event, Bethany returned to the water only a month later, and years later she would end up winning national and international titles. She was only 13 years old when she lost her arm and the majority of her wins were after the incident.

Most athletes are aware that at any moment everything can change. As an athlete, you put quite a bit of emotional and physical toll on your body. Your body is always subject to injury with one wrong move. As a surfer, Bethany was aware that sharks are in the ocean as well as other risks. I don't think Bethany planned on running into a shark that day, but it was a risk she was and continues to take every time she goes into the water. Simply put, something bad happened, she took the necessary time to heal, and she got back up. She accepted what happened and moved on to become one of the most inspiring athletes of the 21st century.

Now I was able to sum up that inspiring story in a short paragraph but I'm sure her journey was anything but short and easy. We are so accustomed to hearing these types of stories over and over that we forget the non-glamorous side of success. We rarely get to see behind the scenes' turmoil that they face. No one wakes up and prepares to lose an arm. You cannot prepare yourself for every possibility to happen in a day. Next, as we talk about preparedness, we are talking about it in a mental sense.

To some degree, we have all had lessons in life that showed us how things can go wrong when we're not prepared. I remember going on a field trip to an arcade-type place in grade school which I anticipated for weeks. Now notice the keyword, ANTICIPATED. I did not plan for the trip. If I had, I wouldn't have left my petty cash at home and spent the whole field trip on the sidelines watching everybody buy games and food while I starved in the corner. If I would have planned ahead, I would have taken my money and placed it by my bookbag to remind me to grab it before leaving for school.

Planning for the future, whether it be for a fun field trip or something more important such as retirement is important. When you plan for things to happen, you are prepared and have an idea or game plan on how to succeed, or at the very least, how to move on from it.

Sometimes life can throw us a curveball, but I would encourage you to expect it. It's not a matter of if something will go wrong in your life, but rather when. These curveballs will vary from person to person and by intensity. Be prepared for setbacks and letdowns, that's life. If you go through life thinking everything should and will go perfectly, you will constantly be in a state of defeat and hopelessness. Life doesn't always go our way but our preparedness will help us embrace these difficult moments and bounce back.

At the same time just because you now know and accept those bad things will happen in life, doesn't mean you spend your time being hopeless and negative. You can try and put yourself in favorable positions to prepare for any emergency, but you also tell yourself that you will tackle any problem when it comes. Trying to imagine every bad thing that can happen will only lead to stress and anxiety. Balance is key here. You cannot control everything in life, but you can fight to make sure that you turn to acceptance and joy when things get bad.

As a fighter, I would go into the ring knowing there was a 100% possibility of me getting hit. Mike Tyson once said, "Everyone knows how to fight until they get punched in the face". For a newbie walking into the ring, getting punched is a shock but most likely there was some probability of that crossing their mind (I mean they're getting in the ring for goodness' sake). However, if you were walking home and someone just punched you out of nowhere you would be completely off guard. They weren't planning on that type of assault.

There is a key difference between planning on something bad happening and anticipating it. I didn't walk into a match anticipating to get hit or to lose. That is how you actually end up losing by the way. But I was prepared in the very least for the opponent to get some hits in. Even the very best fighters in the world get hit during a match. That preparedness of some type of onslaught makes them ask the question "What defense and offense strategy should I use?". That preparedness can give a slight edge over the other opponent if planned right.

At the same time, we don't want to be that person who is just WAITING for the ball to drop. For bad news to be right around the corner. Those are the kinds of people who constantly say things like "I knew I wasn't going to get the job" or "Things were just working out too well, something bad was bound to happen". They anticipate bad news as if they need it to prove something. However, if you chose to plan for things to happen in life, whether enjoyable or bad, you might be a little more inclined to accept and live it fully.

Empowerment comes from knowing that life WILL knock you down, but no matter what making the choice to get back up. You have to mentally prepare yourself to tackle everything that life throws at you. Embrace the difficult times so that you can enjoy the happy ones. Flowers don't grow with sunshine alone; you have to have some rain. Things happen, some you have control over and some you don't. We can accomplish 5 things in a day and if one setback happened, all a sudden we are all out of whack. Plan for things to happen. Plan for LIFE to happen. When things go wrong, it's okay to try to fix it, it's okay to mourn, feel angry, anxious, but we do not want to stay in that state forever. Accepting the fact that something happened does not mean you give up. If you happened to be in an accident and broke your arm you wouldn't just say "This is my life, my arm will always be broken". First, you would get help, that person would pop your arm back into place, then you would take the necessary weeks to heal and move on. This goes the same for accepting other hardships that come with living life. You may seek help, condolement, but eventually, you will need to move on.

So embrace the suck. Life is a giver. It dishes out the good, the bad, and everything in between. Speaking for myself, I do not have psychic abilities, and therefore have no idea when life may take a turn. **The point is to not stress over what MIGHT happen but rather mentally prepare yourself that ANYTHING can happen.** Make a promise to yourself now that no matter what, you will do all you can to get back up when you get knocked down. No one gets out of life alive, but making the most out of your journey will require mental toughness. Sometimes you will have to fight for your joy.

The truth is joyful people know the world is not all sunshine and rainbows. They have not lost touch with reality. They see inequality, poverty, crime, death, and even experience themself. This chapter is so important for you to grasp. You have to make peace with life and all its ugliness. But that does not mean that you have to turn ugly with it. Choose to be that light, that peace, that spark, this world so desperately needs more of. Joyful people are powerful, and you are powerful!

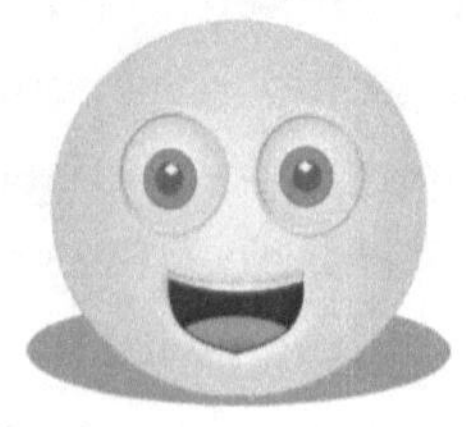

Fun thought: Years ago, I remember coming across a trick that when something doesn't go as planned yell out loud "PLOT TWIST!" I sometimes do it just to bring some humor to the situation. I'll be in line at the grocery store and receive an email saying I owe money. I'll say plot twist and of course, no one will know what I'm talking about but who cares. And yes, saying it out loud makes it that much more impactful and fun.

CH 5: PRACTICE TIME

"If there is something that you want, and you're hungry for it, you've got to do what is required". – Les Brown

Simone Biles made history by becoming the first gymnast to be awarded the most world medals and the most world gold medals.   Her list of accomplishments would take up this whole book so let's just agree that she is pretty great at what she does. Simone trains for 3 hours in the morning and 3 hours in the afternoon. She also cross-trains which includes swimming and riding her bike. Basically, she does what is necessary to be a champion.

You have to make a conscious decision to do what is necessary to live a life of joy. You know life will come with its hardships. You're prepared for whatever life throws at you. Now it's time to learn specifically what you can do every day to CREATE moments of happiness that leads to long-lasting joy. Fortunately, you don't have to wait for the new job or DM reply from your hot crush on Instagram

(@hottieinparadise please message back!). No, you can create your own feelings of happiness without external factors, because joy is developed internally.

Smiling:

First, we are going to start with the physical exercises that lead to feeling happier. Now, this exercise is perfect for people who have a resting b**** face, gotta start working those face muscles more! I was that person that people were constantly asking "Are you okay?" Yes, Julie, this is just my face. It's what I would say but I knew deep down I wasn't happy. Every day I would come into work feeling tired even before 11 am hit. People can see and sense unhappiness even if you don't admit it.

It has been shown that the physical act of smiling can help elevate our mood by triggering the release of neural communication neuropeptides, dopamine, and serotonin. Now I'm not sure what these mood-boosting neurotransmitters are or how to properly pronounce them but they sound like some strong shit! So, skip the coffee in the morning and give yourself a dose of smiles to boost your mood and get you ready for the day.

Smiling is also scientifically proven to be contagious. Not only will you help yourself feel better by smiling, but you may also lead others around you to smile. The area controlling your smiling facial expression is an unconscious automatic response area. Therefore, when people smile at us it is a natural reaction for us to smile back. Ultimately, forced or not, smiling sends the message not only to our brain but to the rest of our body that "Life is good"!

Laughing:

Now this one is my favorite. I get serious "Joker" vibes when doing this exercise. You may have seen this trend on social media where people fake laugh until they start to actually laugh. It's the same concept when practicing happiness. **Fake it until you feel it.**

I have this soft rule of not watching comedy movies and TV shows by myself. I love laughing, it's such a good feeling, but the feeling is even more enjoyable when you have good company to laugh with. You could have graduated high school ten years ago but I bet you still remember the class clown. Humor has a lasting impression.

Laughter is proven to have many benefits when it comes to health in general. Laughter helps release endorphins in our body, which contribute to our feel-good state of being. Endorphins are said to help improve our mood and temporarily reduce pain. Laughter reduces stress by relieving physical tension in the body.

Looking at the funny side of things can also diffuse angry or stressful situations. This can also be a coping mechanism for some people, you can argue at times inappropriately, but that's subjective. Dark humor is very common and popular. Some of the best comedians have dealt with depression and express themselves through comedy. It can help cope or heal even the darkest of situations.

Exercise:

There would be days when I would wake up and realize I have neglected chores, errands, work, etc. due to my 'saddened' state. During those moments I would gather all my resolve and do a hard 50 min run outside. The hotter the better. (Now I know some of you are thinking "50 min ain't nothing, but mind your business, it was hard for me). By the time I got back and took a cold shower, I would be supercharged for the rest of the day. Sometimes we need that feeling of accomplishment of one thing in order to accomplish others. I knew that doing this grueling run would push me to do the other things I didn't want to do.

In track, they used to say, "The hardest part of a run is taking the first step". Once you make the decision to get up and start, things start to fall in place. To get the benefits of exercise, you won't need to train like an athlete. Exercising for even 10 minutes a day will have profound results on your mood compared to no exercise at all. You can choose to run, walk, stretch, swim, etc. Exercising with a friend or in a group setting usually helps to boost your mood.

Mantras:

Now I'm not sure how excited you are about talking to yourself in public, so like laughing this may be something you do in your home. However, if you do start walking around talking about how great you are to no one in particular, I won't judge you. Mantras are positive affirmations about yourself and/or your situation. I was guilty of constantly speaking negative things into existence. I was so used to doing it that it took a friend to point out my behavior and its consequences. I would say things like "I'm so broke" or "I'm just not smart enough". I excused my 'negative talking' as just simply stating facts. I attributed this to the fact that I didn't have a job at the time.

It is true that we are our own worst critics. No one told me I was a failure but that was exactly how I felt. Unfortunately, those thoughts of failure can begin to manifest in negative affirmations. Even when no one was around I would lash out and complain about how incapable I was. In a weird way, I felt as if I deserved the mistreatment for failing. There are things about us that we will want to change, even need to change to be the best version of ourselves. We can be honest about where we are at the moment and envision where we want to be in the future. However, that does not mean constantly repeating about how dumb or weak we are will do us any good.

Positive affirmations can also help to change physical behavior. Building your self-worth will make this exercise much easier and more natural. Just the same, speaking affirmations can help build your self-worth. Truly loving who you are may be difficult for some people, but we eventually want to change that mindset. Since we cannot change our mindset at the snap of our fingers, we will trick our minds by changing our speech.

If you tell yourself that you are worthy and have the ability to reach your goals, then that drive will help you get to that finish line. Speaking positive affirmations is like breathing life into your existence.

Speaking positive affirmations out loud doesn't mean you have to sound like a robot. Actually, saying them in a monotone voice with no enthusiasm or belief will make the success of the exercise even harder. I razzle-dazzle my affirmations with some flare and a few cuss words. Make them you. I can't tell you what to say but these affirmations should make you feel good. You can say them in a funny voice, a coach's tone, or a hype girl voice who only wants the best for you. Clap your hands while you say them, stomp your feet, do a little dance.   Do whatever it takes to help get those affirmations to become beliefs.

Thoughts:

For this exercise, thoughts will be closely correlated to mindfulness.   Being mindful takes practice. Thoughts and feelings arise without our control every day but it's up to us to be mindful by taking into account how we react to them.   It's hard to control our thoughts, especially when they first arise. You can be eating lunch with a friend and all of a sudden wonder if dogs talk about their owners to other dogs behind our backs (the betrayal).

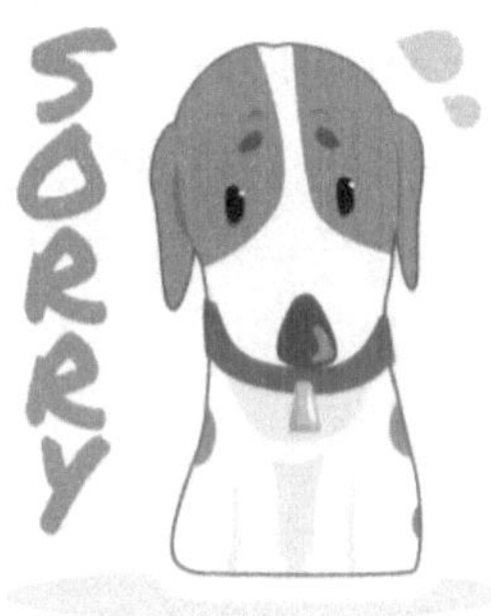

I do not expect you to have every thought that goes through your mind be a positive one. What I will encourage you to do is be mindful when negative thoughts do arise, and then channel positive ones. You may be watching TV and see a really fit actor and think "I'll never look like that". You may have unconsciously come to that conclusion but as you are being mindful of that negative thought, you now chose to replace it with a positive one. Note that positive thoughts do not include putting other people down. So, let's not talk about how that actor has a toned body but their outfit looks like it was picked out in the dark. We're not doing that. #BeNice

Having a high positive to negative thought ratio will improve your overall journey to a more joyful life. It has also been shown that people who tend to be more positive tend to have more friends. Of course, the right friends can lead to more smiles and laughter.

Think back on the previous week of events and point out moments you had negative thoughts. Immediately after, think of the positive attributes that can be associated with those negative thoughts. This can be done on a daily basis also if you're one of the ones who can't even remember what they had for breakfast this morning.

Cold showers:

Ahhh my archnemesis. Although I was born in the Midwest, I have spent the majority of my adult life in Hawaii, and I can 100% be honest and say the thought of willingly taking a cold shower baffled my mind. I used to think "I have worked too hard in life to pretend like I can't afford hot water this month!" No matter, I put my money where my mouth was and decided to just take action and see for myself the benefits that everyone was talking about.

As an athlete, I knew the benefits that ice has on the body. Ice baths help tremendously with muscle recovery after strenuous training. However, you don't have to be an athlete to benefit from cold showers. Stepping into a cold shower helps activate and energize all of your muscles. If continuously done, you will start to see an overall decrease in stress.

A key component from not just getting through the cold showers but also benefiting is by breathing. Think back to the times you are about to jump in a big pool or the ocean. You take a big breath and you don't start breathing again until we break the surface. Mistakenly, most people walk into the cold shower and hold their breath, bracing themselves for the cold onslaught. Taking a big breath at the beginning is important but you want to quickly be able to control your breathing at a slow and steady pace.

Do something you know makes you happy

Most of the previous exercises are done to sort of trick your mind and body into feeling happy. Doing something you like may seem like a no-brainer, but sometimes we need to be reminded to take action when we are feeling down.

Of course, you have to pick a hobby or activity that brings YOU joy. This could be drawing, riding a bike, mediation, photography, dancing, etc. Physically doing something that will help stimulate your body and mind will help boost your mood.

34

CH 6: WHAT'S STOPPING YOU FROM JOY?

Disappointment, negativity, & abuse

What happens when you consistently workout and eat healthy overtime? Well, oftentimes you start to lose weight, gain muscle, lower cholesterol, and overall feel better in the long run. So why doesn't everyone do that when they are looking for those types of results? The truth is change requires work and that work has to come from you. Some people shy away from hard work as it can be very uncomfortable. Think of any successful athlete or business person. They do whatever needs to be done to get the outcome they desire. The process may be simple but it's never easy.

Sometimes negative and hurtful people can make it difficult to be in a joyful state. Some of you are surrounded by negativity, people claiming they know who you are and what you are capable of. You may have grown up hearing that you are just an angry person, that's just who you are. Or you may have been neglected, laughed at, looked over again and again. Others may have experienced physical abuse. Life itself may have dealt you blow after blow, and now you wonder if you will ever be happy.

Michael Jordan, arguably the greatest basketball player to ever live, went to accomplish many feats as a player for the Chicago Bulls. As an inspired sophomore in high school, Jordan went to try out for the varsity basketball team. Unfortunately, he did not make the team and ended up being put on the JV team. Michael was crushed and went home to cry in his room when he found out the news. Everyone has a choice to make after life seems to halt our dreams or take something special away. We can continue crying and believe in our shortcomings or we can do everything in our power to prove them wrong.

That season Michael trained rigorously, visualizing his spot on the varsity team next year. He ended up excelling on the JV team that year and making it to the varsity team the following year as he envisioned. That driven mentality to work for what you want led Michael to become one of the greatest athletes of all time. You have the choice to allow outside opinions to dictate who you are or you can build yourself into the person that you want to be.

Toxic relationships are like heavy chains weighing you down. Abusive relationships can not only be negative but also deadly. Leaving them is not always easy especially if you are dependent on that individual. Make sure you talk with someone you trust and create a plan to safely leave the situation. Living in these types of relationships will have you in a constant state of anxiety, stress, and fear. It will be nearly impossible to live a life of joy in these situations. If you cannot leave the situation immediately due to the factor the hurtful people may be family or a partner, do your best to find someone you trust and can talk to. In these difficult situations, it is always important to have a friend, counselor, or network to provide resources and support.

Milestone happiness

For most people, living a life of joy is hindered due to their own limitations and beliefs. At an early age, we are programmed to hit milestones and then celebrate them. We are given a vague map of what to do in order to be successful. Some of these common milestones include, graduate high school, go to college, make good money, own a home, and retire early.

Success doesn't have to mean making a million dollars or winning a gold medal at the Olympics. There is no milestone you have to hit to prove to people that you made it. Besides, these examples of success do not correlate to happiness. You can build a wealthy empire and still feel scared and alone. If we want to really succeed, we have to find joy. That joy does not come from external forces such as prizes, money, jobs, recognition, and material things. Joy is cultivated internally by making peace with who you are and where you are at that moment.

Self-sabotage

Not all of us have those external forces undermining our capabilities. Self-sabotage, drama seekers, comfort zones, can all assist in limiting your ability to thrive. There are many ways you can exhibit self-sabotaging behavior. Some examples include comparing yourself to other people, doing activities that you know will make you even sadder or angry, indulging in alcohol or drugs, or quitting.

When things get difficult, we tend to fall back on our old habits because they are what we are used to. Those suffering from addictions are at their most vulnerable state when stressed or upset, as they may relapse. Self-sabotaging behaviors are habits and can be hard to break. This is especially due to the fact that they usually make you feel good in the short-term but will have a negative effect in the long-term.

There are also people who feel the need to have some type of drama going on in their life. If there isn't drama, they'll make some up. If you are that person who spreads rumors, gossips, takes on unnecessary risks, indulges in unhealthy behaviors, you probably already know you have to make a change. Chances are you've seen what your destructive behaviors and thoughts have done to yourself and others. It's time to examine those behaviors and thoughts and find out what's fueling them. Ultimately, you are the one who has to change them and see the benefits of doing so.

You may be surprised to believe that some people no matter how miserable, are comfortable with their misery. Fear of change is real no matter if that change is for the better. You may see how what you're doing is destructive and still not be willing to change. We've all heard the saying "You can lead a horse to water but you can't make him drink". Fear of breaching outside your comfort zone may stem from disappointment, loss of hope, or ignorance.

You have to get uncomfortable with yourself. No longer should you be comfortable with your destructive behavior and negative thoughts. It takes strength to face your demons every day, but a strong enough drive of something better will help you tackle any hardships.

I used to do some of the same destructive behaviors because it was what I was used to. I would know what I was doing was counterproductive to the joyful life I wanted to live. However, setbacks allowed me to lose hope of truly reaching my goal. Sometimes we get tired of trying but know this: What doesn't kill you makes you stronger. But that doesn't happen on its own. You have to choose to get stronger. Keep fighting, and don't give up, because the only real failure is actually giving up" -Jocko Willink

Ultimately, what is stopping you from living a life full of joy is yourself. Opening yourself up to joy is a necessary step to allowing other opportunities that you never thought was possible to enter your life. **Joy brings hope, and hope gives you the strength to overcome any obstacle and any person.**

CONCLUSION: PRACTICE LIKE YOUR LIFE DEPENDS ON IT

*"I fear not the man who has practiced
10,000 kicks once but fear the man who
has practiced one kick 10,000 times"*
- Bruce lee

Repetition is vital in elite training. Trainers and coaches know the importance of adding it into training plans and have seen positive results from it. When I would do private lessons for boxing, I would often get those students who always wanted to move on to the next thing. I get it, you pay someone to teach you, and now you expect to use every minute of that hour learning as much as you can. They didn't know that I would have days in training that all we would throw is the jab, the first punch you learn in boxing. Hard work is not always glamorous. You have to do the work people don't want to do.

If you want to be good at something, you have to practice over and over. Like an athlete there will be moments that you won't want to do them. Make these exercises become habits so that these feelings of happiness come more naturally. You will start to find yourself doing them even when you aren't sad. It will no longer be a survival mechanism of getting you out of dark places, but rather a daily routine of conscious living.

Freedom from your emotions is such a liberating thing. External factors no longer have to define your state of joy. You can choose when to feel happy by practicing the mentioned exercises.

Notice the theme of the book deals with choice. If you choose not to be happy, you are mostly hurting yourself. Family and friends will be affected by your decision but it's you who will suffer the most.

Remember the story about David Goggins and his 100-mile test to run in the Badwater Ultramarathon? Later when he completed the test people would ask him if it was his family or fellow service members that drove him to complete the race. It wasn't. It was personal. He was so driven to push his mind and body to the limit to become the greatest person that he could be. And you have to do the same thing. You have to start this journey for yourself, and do all the hard work that comes with it.. Don't treat joy as this thing that may come if you're lucky. Demand happiness in your life, you're worth it.

Making the decision to live a life of joy is not enough. You need to take action. Do these daily exercises laid out in the book consistently for a month before you ever think about giving up. These conscious decisions to improve your mood will soon become unconscious habits. You owe it to yourself to be filled with joy and surrounded by positivity. It is never too late to transform your life. So, get up, smile, laugh, sweat, dance, talk, do whatever it takes to feel happy and live a life of joy!

The Sport of Happiness:

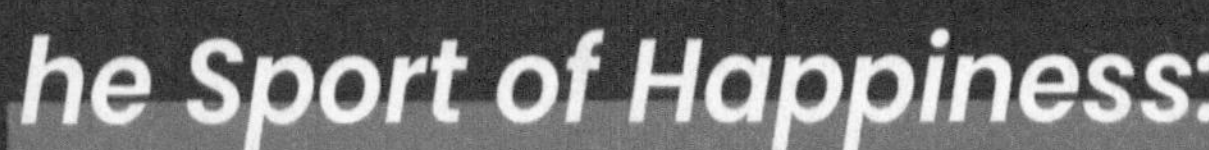

Playbook

Reflection & Exercises to Help Turn Knowledge Into Action

By: Iasha King

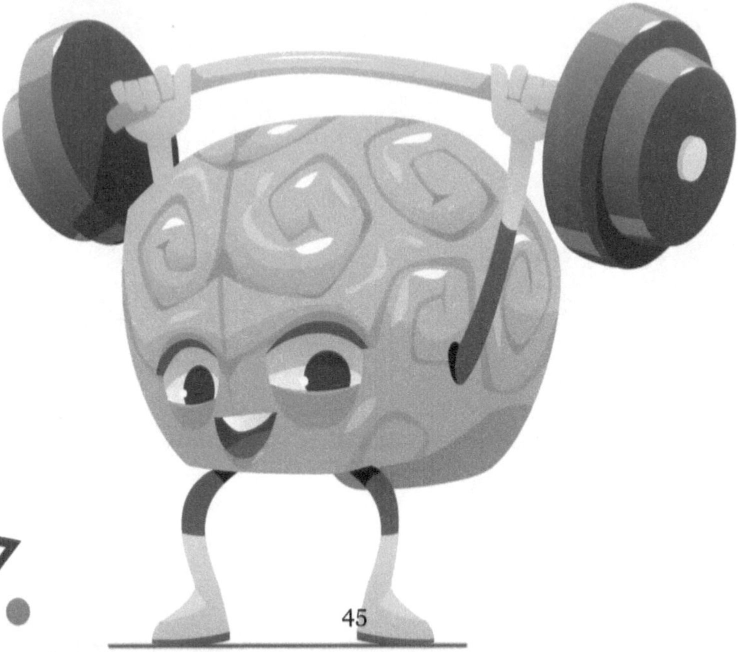

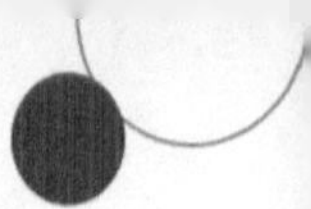

I'm so glad that you took the time to download this playbook to go along with "The Sport of Happiness". There will be a Journal/Reflect section as well as a Practice section for each chapter. The journaling will help you learn something new about yourself and the practice section will help build what we call 'happiness habits'.

I encourage you to have a separate notebook for journaling. This is no test and will not be shared with anyone else, so be very honest with yourself when answering.

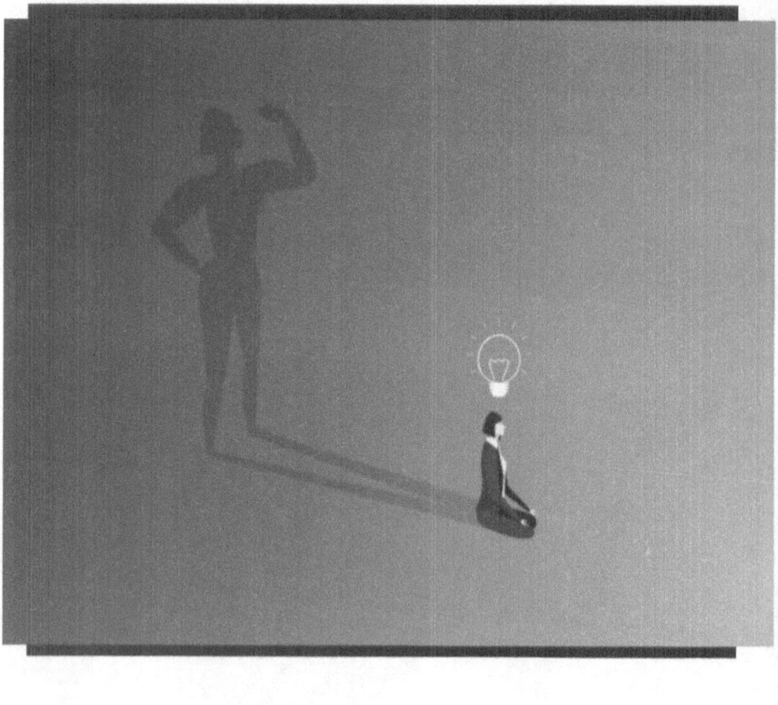

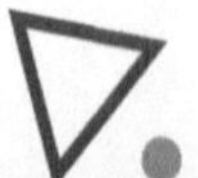

Hello World!

The journal that telss all my secrets and deepest thoughts. Keep out

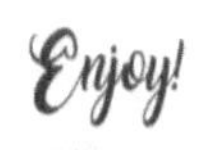

Feelings Are Tricky

You've learned that feelings aren't always what they seem, and can arise when we least expect them. The biggest mistake is letting those feelings stop us from achieving our goals. If we want to lose 20 pounds, the feeling of laziness may stop us from getting the necessary exercise. If we want to save money, feeling the need to keep 'appearances' by buying material things will stop us from saving adequately. You must see feelings as temporary states of emotions and work on not allowing them to dictate your action.

Journal & Reflect:

1. What is a goal you made for yourself recently that fell through? What were some of the feelings that stopped you from working/achieving your goal?

2. Laziness is often the reason we are unable to hit our goals. What have you sacrificed by being lazy?

Practice:

1. Try to point out your feelings throughout the day for 10 days. Notice when you are anxious, upset, stressed, sad, etc. In the future, it will be important to identify the triggers and negative behaviors that may consequently follow.

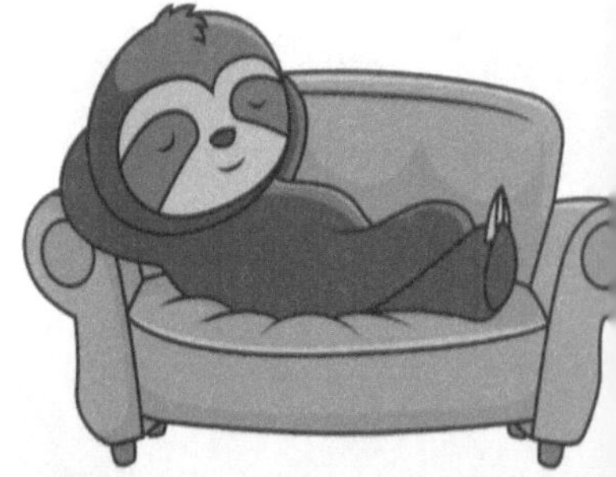

Remember to not ignore your feelings as they come. Later in the book, you will learn to be mindful of these feelings and eventually acknowledge and accept them as they are. This does not mean acting out on them. Say an event happens that leads to you feeling anger. Just because you feel a sudden rise of anger does not mean you now have to act out on that anger. You will begin to understand that you have more power over your emotions than you think.

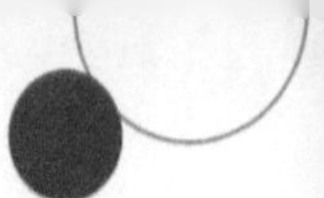
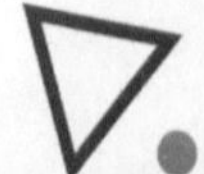

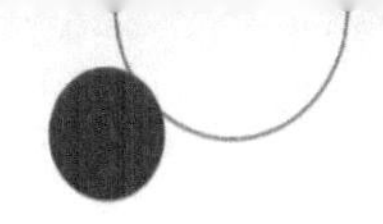

JOURNAL & REFLECT

Feelings Are Tricky

on't forget- no one else sees the world the way you do, so no one else can tell the stories that you have to tell" - Charles de Lint

NAME

DATE

JOURNAL & REFLECT

Continued Writing Space

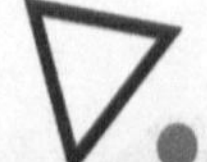

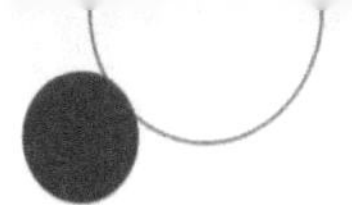

Pain & Perspective

We know pain is real, and that no one should fault us for having human emotion. We have our wins and losses every day. Despite these challenges that life may bring, it should never stop us from practicing gratefulness. Gratefulness helps us to become empathetic, more positive, and at peace with ourselves.

Journal & Reflect:

Reflect back to a time where something bad happened to you and you became extremely upset, but that bad moment turned into something good in the future. Example: Losing a job but finding another with a higher salary and better work environment.

Practice:

At the end of every night right down something you are grateful for. Again, this does not have to be something big. Do this for 10 days straight.

Recycle your pain by turning it into something positive. This could be as simple as you acknowledge that 'life happens' and move forward.

During a certain period of my life, I felt that my life was very dull and boring. I had shelter, food, a job, friends, and more, but I didn't really feel that happy most of the time. So I started this project where I would buy those big yearly print calendars. Instead of using that calendar for planning, I used that calendar to write down something I did or that I was grateful for that day. Some of those days were filled with adventure, other days were just grateful statements. It was nice being able to reflect and see all the things I was actually doing in life and what I had. I encourage you to place your gratefulness highlights where you can see them.

7.

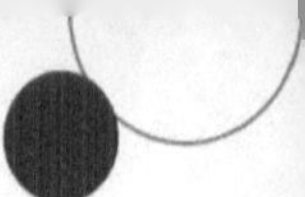

JOURNAL & REFLECT

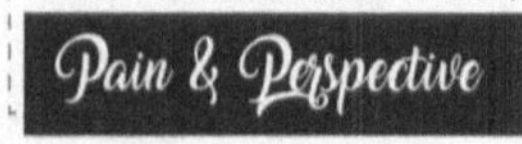

"You don't have to control your thoughts. You just have to stop them fro

controlling you"- Dan Millman

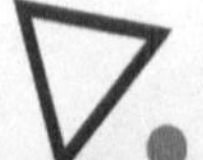

JOURNAL & REFLECT

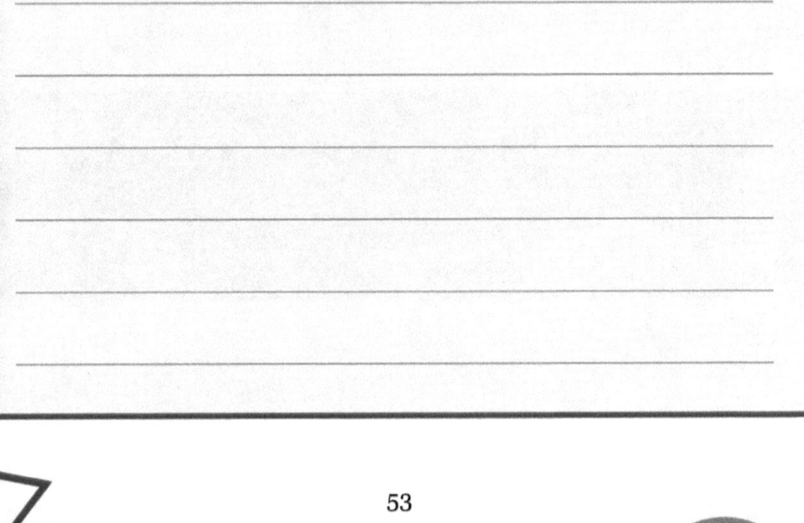

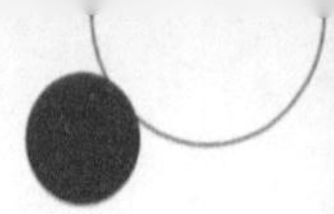

Happiness vs. Joy

Remember, a joyful life is the end goal. Happiness is volatile, dependent on external events, people, material gain, etc. There is nothing wrong with feeling happy but we do not want to wait on these external forces to give us permission to be happy. With joy, we allow ourselves to have internal peace. We don't want to get in the habit of 'milestone happiness'. That is telling yourself that you will be happy once blank happens.

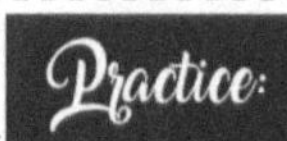

1. What are some short and long-term goals you have for yourself? How have you been feeling and treating yourself in the meantime?

2. Reflect back on your life and see if there was a time you felt joy for a long period of time. What do you think was the cause of that?

Practice:

1. Celebrate the small wins every day for 10 days. That could be giving yourself a pat on the back for waking up early. Or one day going out to eat for submitting your application to grad school.

Allowing joy to enter our lives does not hinder our ability to strive to be better people. Although we may accept where we are today by being joyful, we can still be driven to work towards a better tomorrow. Being joyful does not mean you are out of touch with reality. You can be truthful with yourself, informed of what is going on around you, without being persuaded by it.

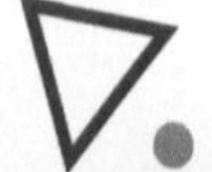

NAME ______________ DATE ______________

JOURNAL & REFLECT

Happiness Vs. Joy

"Never give up on things that make you smile"

NAME

DATE

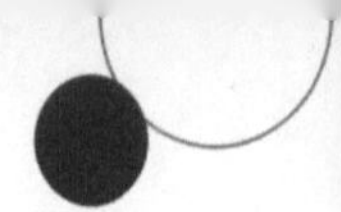

JOURNAL & REFLECT

Continued Writing Space

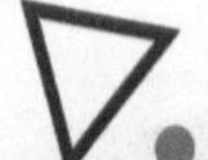

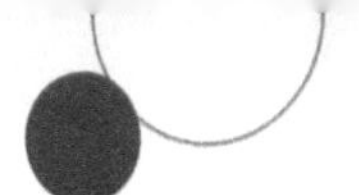

Embrace the Suck

Hardships will come your way and bad things are going to happen to everyone. While we don't say that to be negative, we do point this out so that you are prepared to fall, but that you promise to get back up. Going back to our section on feelings. Feeling sad after a loved one passes away is normal. However, staying in that state of mourning can be detrimental if staying for too long. Striving for a joyful life can sometimes feel like a fight. It's hard, you have forces fighting against you, but you must continue to push forward.

Journal & Reflect:

Is there a moment in your life where you thought you wouldn't be able to continue? If so, what brought you out of your dark place?

Hard work requires sacrifice. What sacrifices have you made in order to reach your goals? Have they worked?

Practice:

Now that you plan on life happening (the good and the bad) the next time something happens that doesn't go your way, accept it as it is and strive to move on.

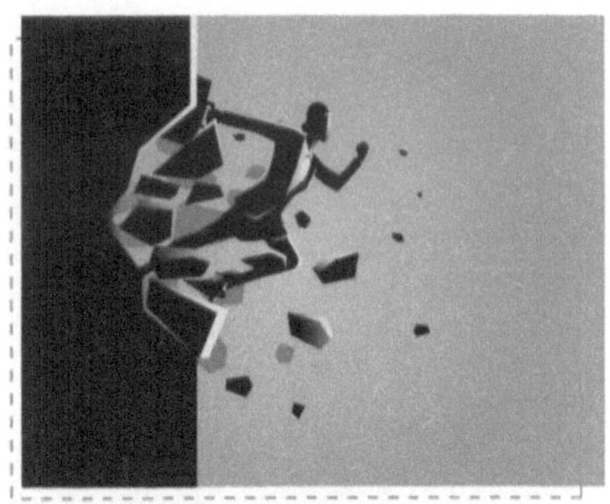

Recycle your pain. Don't just go through something difficult and let that be it. Learn from it and grow from it. Check out this amazing story of boxer, Buster Douglass and his defeat against Mike Tyson. It still gives me chills to this day. Joy requires resilience. Watch **HERE**

7.

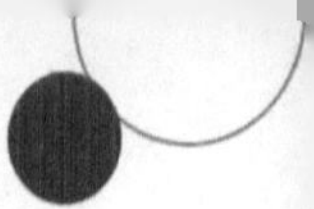

NAME _______________   DATE _______________

JOURNAL & REFLECT

Embrace The Suck

"It's okay to be a glowstick; sometimes we need to break before we shin

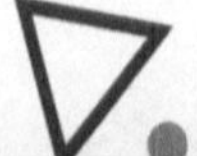

JOURNAL & REFLECT

Continued Writing Space

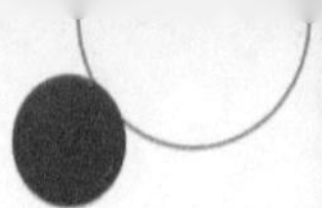

Practice Time

Now you have the exact tools laid out for you. These exercises will help trick your body and mind into thinking you are happy, giving you an immediate feeling of happiness. There are various forms of exercise, some will work better for you than others. It's up to you to find out which one works best. You are putting power back into your hands. You're not waiting for milestones to be reached or material things. You decide when you want to feel happy.

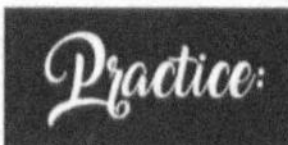

Journal & Reflect:

1. Before actually starting to practice these exercises, which ones do you think will work best for you?

Practice:

1. Now that you have practiced being mindful of your emotions. The next time you feel angry or sad, take a moment to do one or multiple exercises. Do this consistently for 30 days!

Smiling:

- Smile really big (over exaggerate, the crazier you look the better) 10 times. Afterward, you will feel your face start to relax. Then take the next step in relaxing your body and thoughts.

- Long-term: When you wake up in the morning try holding a smile for a whole minute. Hold a good posture while you do this whether that's standing or sitting

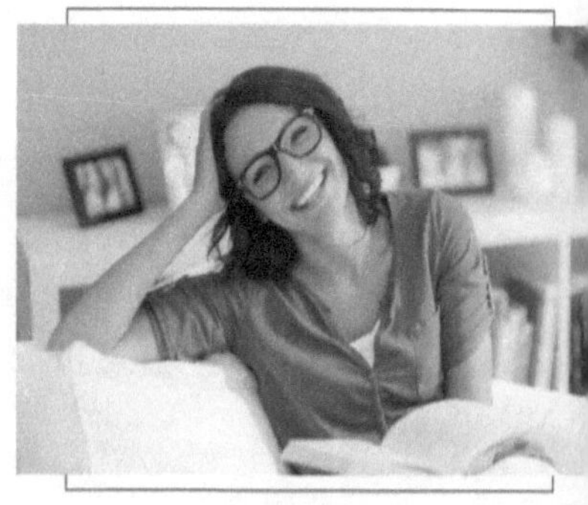

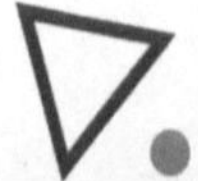

NAME

DATE

JOURNAL & REFLECT

Practice Time

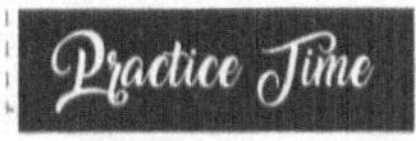

"Think progress not perfection"

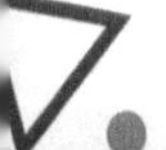

NAME

DATE

JOURNAL & REFLECT

Continued Writing Space

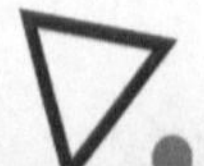

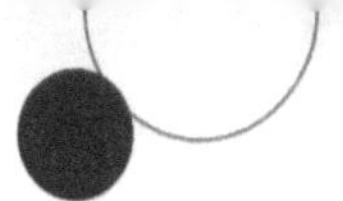

Laughing:

- Do your own version of the Tik Tok challenge by laughing until you feel better. If you have to make a card that explains your "situation" when you choose to do it outside, by all means, go for it (another "Joker" reference for those unable to keep up).

- Long-term hack: Instead of running to sad music or a dark room to cry yourself to sleep, try putting on a clip or show that will put a smile on your face or make you laugh.

Exercise:

- Do a hard workout. Of course, this is subjective to you, just make sure you push yourself.

- Long-term: Make exercise a daily or weekly habit by implementing time in your schedule. Stick to it even when you may not feel like it.

> *Hack: Find a workout partner to hold you accountable and make it fun

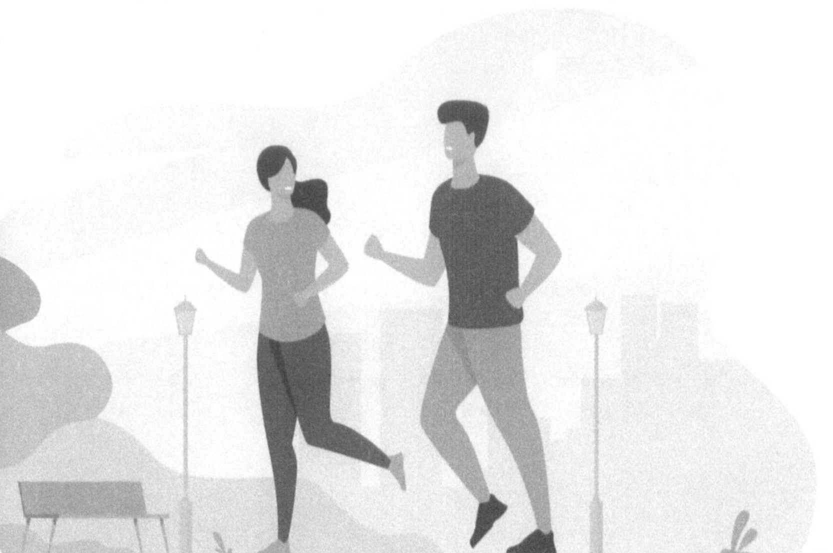

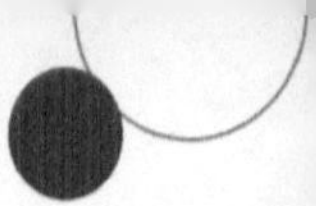

Mantras:

- Speak positive affirmations in regards to what you are feeling. For example, if you are feeling frustrated about not understanding course material, say things like "I will get this" or acknowledge "This is difficult but one day I will understand".

- Long-term: Speak positive affirmations towards other people also. The positive talk should be a part of our daily life and should encourage those around us.

Thoughts:

- Immediately after a negative thought comes to mind, think of something positive. The positive attributes do not have to be big.

- Long-term: Work on building your sense of self-worth and believe in your capabilities. We wouldn't allow someone to slander the ones we love. In the same respect, we shouldn't allow ourselves to be slandered.

Cold showers:

- Whenever you are feeling down in general, these cold showers will sharpen you up really quickly. Make sure you are breathing in and out at a steady pace. Start out for a short duration of about 1-2 minutes and then gradually up your time to about 10 min/day.

- Some people chose to take a cold shower every day. Find a time/day(s) in your schedule to fit in this exercise regularly.

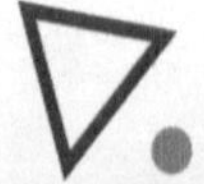

Positive

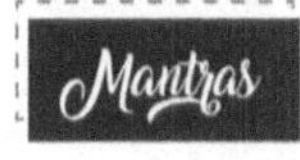

1.

2.

3.

4.

5.

6.

7.

8.

9.

10.

Say Them Throughout The Day

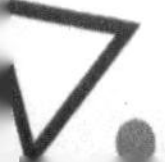

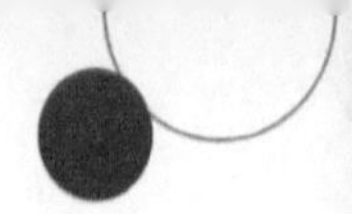

Do something that makes you happy:

- Choose a hobby or activity that has brought you a feeling of happiness or ease in the past. This should calm you down immediately.

- Long-term: Learning something new can be an exciting time for most people. If you feel stuck in a rut try joining a new class or train for something new. You will feel challenged, exhilarated, and will hopefully bring more feelings of joy.

To start off your 30-day joy challenge, make sure you implement some of the above exercises into your daily routine. Hang this planner on a wall where you can easily see it every day. Don't allow yourself to skip items during this 30-day practice. Here is an example of how you can implement the new daily exercises.

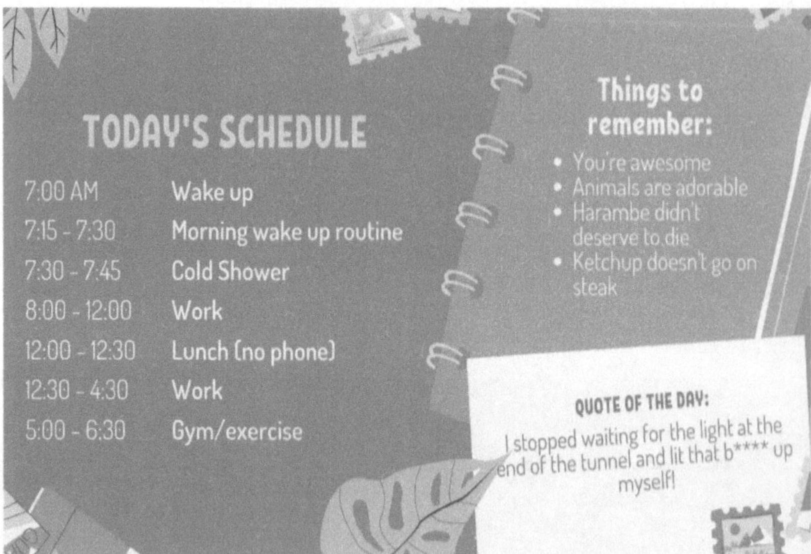

You should feel a slight improvement in your mood after doing an exercise. However, the more you consistently practice, the more likely they will become habits. Eventually, it will not be as hard to stop and change your mood. You will start to see the benefits and want to implement them even when you don't feel sad or angry.

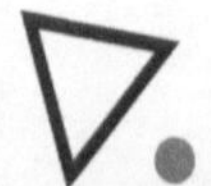

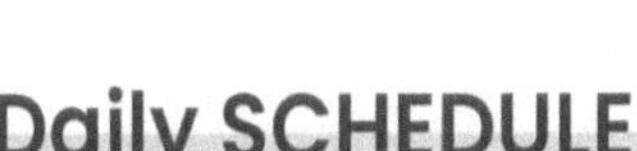

Daily SCHEDULE

6 AM

7 AM

8 AM

9 AM

10 AM

11 AM

12 PM

1 PM

2 PM

3 PM

4 PM

5 PM

TODAY'S TASKS

What is Stopping You From Being Happy?

Whether it's self-sabotage or external forces making your joy journey difficult, you must make the decision to let them go.

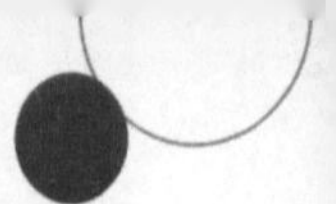

Journal & Reflect:

1. Identify self-sabotaging behaviors that you have

2. Write down their short-term effects and long-term consequences

3. Who are people you feel are negatively impacting your life?

4. How do you plan on removing yourself from them?

5. On a scale of 1-10, how committed are you in implementing these 'happiness habits' (10 being most committed)?

Practice:

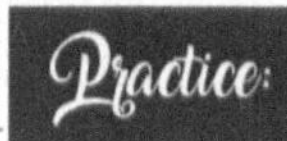

1. In every area of your life start taking action. Doing what is necessary should become a habit.

Self-discipline is another component of your joy journey. If you had a goal of losing 15 pounds but realized you only lost 2 pounds in the past 30 days would you quit? Some people would, others would be even more driven to keep going. Find what works and stick with it. You may not see long-lasting results immediately but long-lasting results require long-lasting practice!

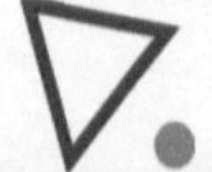

JOURNAL & REFLECT

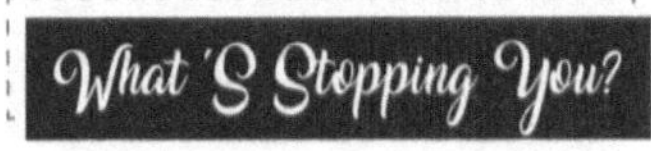

Trust in the magic of new beginnings"

NAME

DATE

JOURNAL & REFLECT

Continued Writing Space

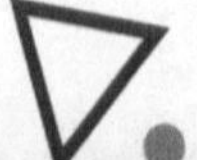

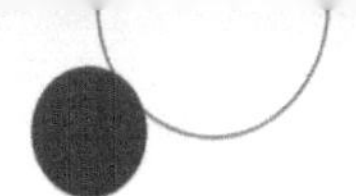

Next Steps

Do it!

That's it, just take action. You may slack off or indulge in self-sabotaging behavior here and there but don't give up. If you quit working on yourself you will never change.

We all need an open community where we can be ourselves, ask questions, and meet amazing people. Make sure you follow our Facebook page to learn about resources available to you and events that may be going on in your area. We will also be starting a group soon where everyone can share their journey, connect, and learn from each other.

To follow our Facebook page and join the community check us out at:
Facebook.com/socialhumanpublishing

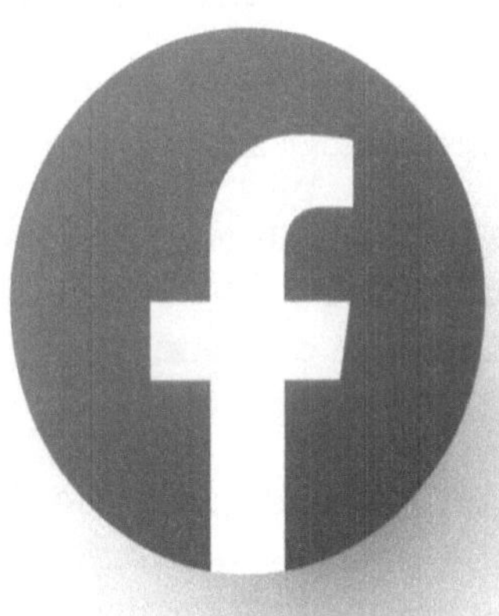

Stay tuned for our upcoming releases! Feel free to contact us at any time. We are a small team of authors and contributors and are excited to meet you and hear about your journey!

Email: aloha@socialhumanpub.com

REFERENCES:

Farah, A. F. (2016, June 29). *Olympian Simone Biles Dishes on How She's Training, Eating, and Mentally Prepping Before Rio*. Women's Health Magazine. https://www.womenshealthmag.com/fitness/a19982193/simone-biles-rio-olympics/

Flax, P. F. (2008, October 24). *The Warrior: David Goggins*. Runners World. https://www.runnersworld.com/runners-stories/a20798013/rw-hero-of-running-david-goggins/

Hof, W. (2020). The Wim Hof Method: Activate Your Full Human Potential. United States: Sounds True.

Joy vs. Happiness. (2015, September 1). Psychologies. https://www.psychologies.co.uk/joy-vs-happiness

Kennedy, T. K. (2011, December 18). *The Power of Perspective*. HuffPost. https://www.huffpost.com/entry/positive-attitude-advice_b_1018175

Laughter is the Best Medicine. (2020, October). Help Guide. https://www.helpguide.org/articles/mental-health/laughter-is-the-best-medicine.htm

Marmolejo-Ramos, F., Murata, A., Sasaki, K., Yamada, Y., Ikeda, A., Hinojosa, J. A., Ospina, (2020, February 4). Your face and moves seem happier when I smile. Facial action   influences the perception of emotional faces and biological motion stimuli. https://doi.org/10.31234/osf.io/4uvdq

Rao, C. R. (2020, March 14). *Was Michael Jordan
     Really Cut From His High School Basketball Team?*
     Sports Casting.
     https://www.sportscasting.com/was-michael-
     jordan-really-cut-from-his-high-school-basketball-
     team/

Reynolds, G. R. (2018, March 2). *Even a Little Exercise
     Might Make Us Happier*. The New York Times.
     https://www.nytimes.com/2018/05/02/well/move/
     even-a-little-exercise-might-make-us-happier.html

Ruby, F. J. M., Smallwood, J., Engen, H., & Singer, T.
     (2013). How self-generated thought shapes mood—
     The relation between mind-wandering and mood
     depends on the socio-temporal content of
     thoughts. *PLoS ONE, 8*(10), Article
     e77554. https://doi.org/10.1371/journal.pone.00775
     54

Stibich, M. S. (2020, February 23). *The Benefits of
     Positive Thinking and Happiness*. Very Well Mind.
     https://www.verywellmind.com/accentuate-the-
     positive-positive-thinking-and-happiness-

Using Affirmations. (2021). Mind Tools.
     https://www.mindtools.com/pages/article/affirmati
     ons.htm

Wood, A., Rychlowska, M., Korb, S., & Niedenthal, P.
     (2016). Fashioning the face:
     Sensorimotor simulation contributes to facial
     expression recognition. *Trends in Cognitive
     Sciences, 20*(3), 227–
     240. https://doi.org/10.1016/j.tics.2015.12.010